WHAT'S HAPPENING TO ME NOW?!

THE FACTS OF LIFE, AS A WOMAN IN YOUR ~~20S~~ 40S. (STRAIGHT TALK ABOUT PERIMENOPAUSE.)

Written by Heather Wright

Illustrated by Matylda McCormack-Sharp

For all the sweating, exhausted, outraged women, everywhere.

And for the mere mortals trying to support them.

ISBN-9781970109245
First printing: 2020

Printed in the United States of America

This book is for you, lovely.

Yes, **YOU.** (The one panicking.)

The one suffering from yet another of life's hormonally **CRAZY** phases.

Without enough helpful information about what it is. And if anything can be done about it.

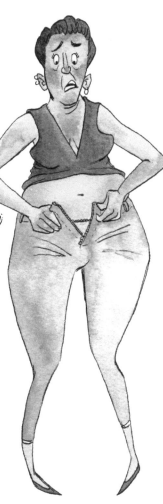

PERI....WHAT?!

There you are, lying with your legs spread eagle, your exposed lady parts swinging in the brisk air of your lovely obstetrician's office for an annual exam, when BANG! The word is casually released like an advanced nuke dropped from the B-2 stealth bomber... **PERIMENOPAUSE.** Okay, breathe. All women go through it. But this idea of "going through puberty backward" (go on, whisper it... *menopause*) is, t a b o o. We simply don't want to talk about it! Or we whisper together, exposing ourselves to grapevine-style misinformation. There was an array of perfectly reasonable looking books and articles on the market; but nothing like what I wanted. I was searching for a short, sweet, and humorous explanation of what the hell was going on with my body, and if there was anything I could immediately do about it. You know, now that we can finally admit that we aren't 29-years-and-holding. I'd like to tell you that your doctor could guide you through it all. (Just wait until you find out what little data that esteemed character is operating on.) I'm not going to sugar coat this; there may be perplexing years ahead. This book cannot answer all of your questions. Hint: There aren't always answers. It is not a substitute for medical advice or clinical research (as if there were much of that available, ladies). My humble aim is that you may be better positioned to find an approach that works for you, or at least that we share some good old-fashioned laughter to ease the uncomfortable bits.

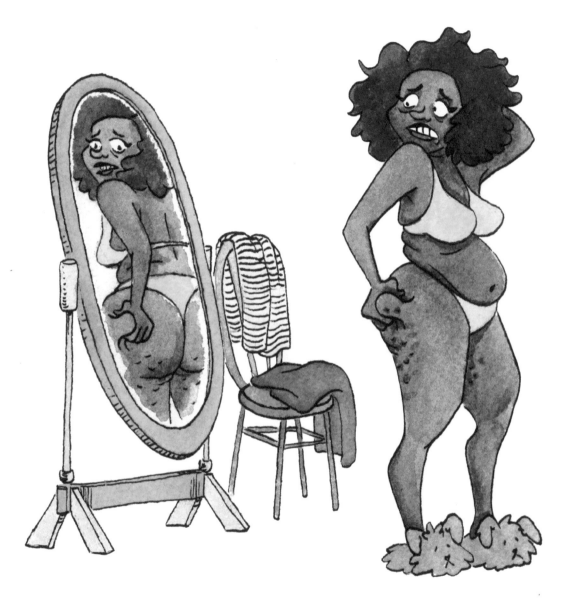

It's not a shock that you don't want to know.

MYTHS

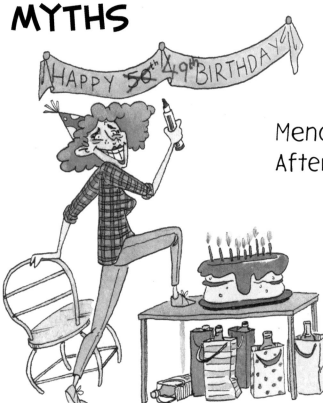

Menopause happens overnight.
After I'm 50.

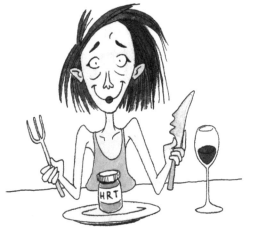

Hormone replacement therapy
(HRT) will stop the nonsense!

I will have symptoms. Forever.

I'll have no sex life (...ever again).

Surgery means I skip
the symptoms.

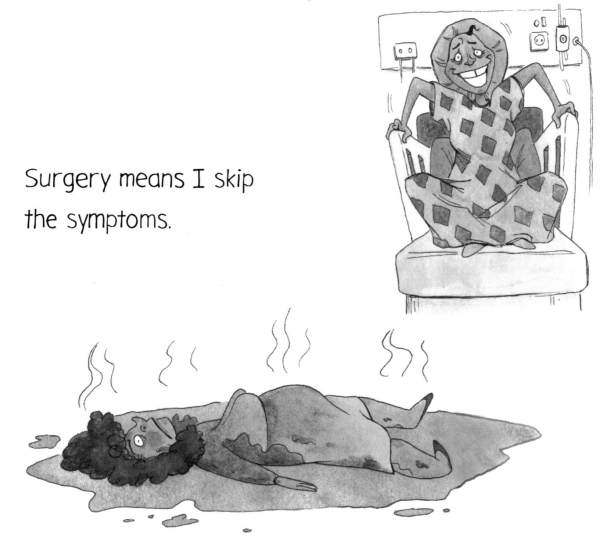

I'm doomed to gain weight and drown in a pool of sweat.

WHY THE TABOO?

So why the myths? The subject is **TABOO.** *So let's talk about it!* Quietly. In many cultures, youth is desirability. Often there are no defined roles for older women. If menopause signals the end of youth and perceived value and we don't know what comes after, is it surprising nobody wants to talk about it? Some women lament the end of their child-bearing days, including women who may have tried everything to get pregnant and may be facing the hard reality that the trying is over. Is it any wonder that you run screaming "Not Me!"

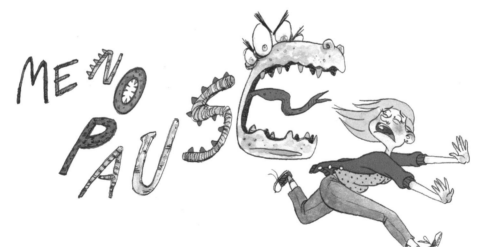

The role and status of women during their fertile years are seen to reverse at menopause. Rates of reported psychological symptoms vary across cultures. Distress is reported high for Jewish American women. It is low for women from India of the royal Rajput "caste" whose lives gain more freedom after menopause.[1]

A taboo subject can mean less access to facts supporting informed decisions. According to Dr. P. Mansfield, educated women are informed by friends, books, media, mothers, sit-coms (!)...the last resort is a doctor.[2] It can be difficult for some women to open up about symptoms. It may not be clear that some symptoms are related to changing hormone levels. The least likely subject a woman will bring to their gynecologist is about a change in sexual interest.[3] When one woman turns to another for advice, misinformation can be passed on.

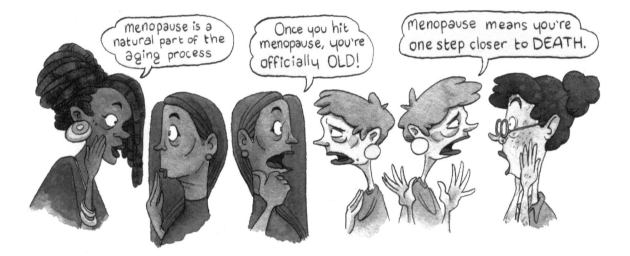

Even more dangerous than prevailing cultural attitudes is a shameful lack of research funding.[4] Women's health has taken the lowest priority in American governmental studies and research grants.[5] American national research institutes have perpetuated women's state of ignorance about menopause because there is a significant ongoing bias across healthcare studies that renders women almost invisible in the data.[6] So what data do you think your doctor is using to guide you?

WHY MENOPAUSE?

Menopause comes from two Greek words (but it's not their fault, so be nice).

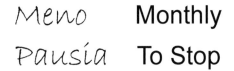

Meno	Monthly
Pausia	To Stop

That's it! Menopause is the cessation of your monthly period. But not your life, okay? Twelve consecutive months without menstruating is post-menopausal. But you don't just leap to it! More about stages in a minute.

Before you start howling in protest, briefly consider why this is useful. Babies are hard work; to birth and to raise! Apes do not have menopause. If the ape mother lives a long time, it is possible that she will die when her last baby is still dependent on her. In that case, according to the esteemed Jane Goodall, the baby usually dies too. Mothers need to be young to handle the rigors of birthing and the high demands of child-rearing.[7] You caught me, I'm speculating. Before I get a lot of hate mail from a host of involved grandparents rearing grandchildren, it should be recognized that plenty of grandparents in history have stepped up to raise a baby quite well, thank you very much. I'm simply postulating that this is Mother Nature's clever approach to help the human tribe. Silver linings, anyone?

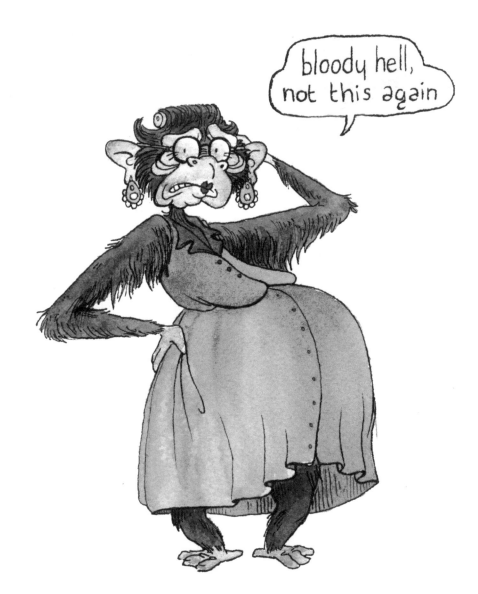

"It's the tragedy of [female apes] having no menopause. The last child is likely to die because the mother is too old to provide proper nutrition."

- Jane Goodall[8]

A JOURNEY

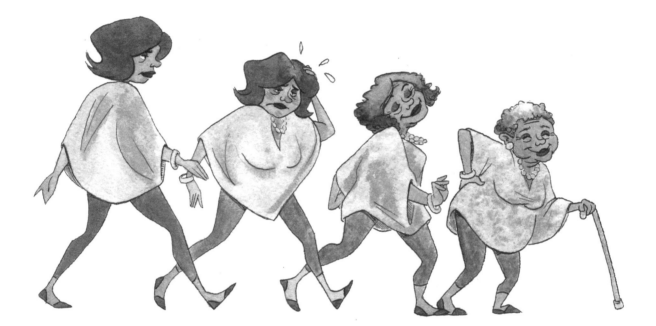

I liked the way Gail Sheehy breaks the post-reproductive life into four stages[9]:

1. **Perimenopausal**   Start of the transition (bloody uncomfortable, pun intended).
2. **Menopause**   Completion of the ovarian transition, 1 year–no period.
3. **Coalescence**   'Post-Menopausal Zest.'
4. **Maturescence**   Passage into full maturity in the 70s.

When changes start to happen, and it's sooner than you think, it may be hard to even recognize it, never mind adjust. The process may take longer than expected.

Onset. Research shows it's far earlier than we thought. For many women, this can mean the late 30s.

The ovarian transition is the acute period of biological passage, spanning five to seven years. This is the rough part, ladies. This often happens from age 47 or 48 to the mid-50s.

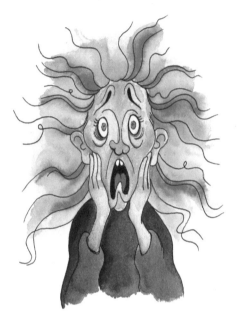

For perhaps three years (let's say 48 to 51 years-ish) for women with an intact uterus, the female body is just out of sync with its own chemistry.

While the average age of natural menopause is 51, in the U.S., there are reasons why a woman can go through it earlier. Causes of "premature menopause" can include genetics, illness, or medical procedures (e.g., hysterectomy, removal of ovaries). About a third of women between 25 to 44 years in the U.S. reach menopause through surgery. These women experience twice as many depressive symptoms than any other group.[10]

WHAT TO EXPECT: SYMPTOMS

There is a dramatic reduction in estrogen and progesterone, the reproductive hormones, during aging. Dr. Jen Gunter explains that "the ability of the follicles to produce estrogen declines, so the brain produces higher levels of follicle-stimulating hormone in an attempt to stimulate the ovaries... it's as if the brain keeps shouting at the ovaries to produce estrogen, and there is no mechanism for the ovaries to reply."[11] Symptoms are not linked to hormone levels, but to genetics, tolerance, and estrogen stored in fat.

Wait, **SYMPTOMS...?**

10-15% of women report no problems with menopause

15% of women are rendered temporarily dysfunctional

70% of women wrestle with symptoms associated with menopause[12]

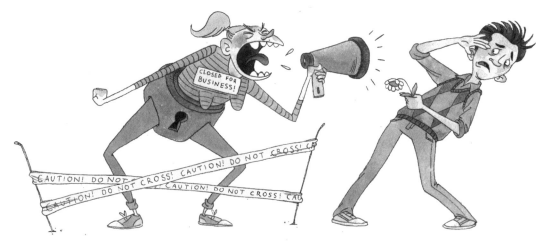

Gushing (sudden heavy flow of blood), erratic periods

Changes in libido, decreased sexual response

"Electrical surges", electrical sensation, tingling of skin

Heart disease, palpitations, racing

Weight gain

Cysts in breasts

Fibroid mass in uterus

Hot flashes, night sweats

Skin changes (e.g., papery, leathery)

Osteoporosis, bone loss, bone fractures

Vaginal atrophy, pain, dryness

Bladder incontinence

Joint Muscle Pain

Numbness in hands and feet

Memory loss

Lower mental acuity

Difficulty concentrating

Static in the brain

Headaches, migraines

Fatigue, loss of energy, trouble sleeping

Mood swings (sharp temper, anyone?)

Anxiety, depression (can't shake the blues)

Restlessness

Self-destructive behaviors (e.g., affairs, drugs)

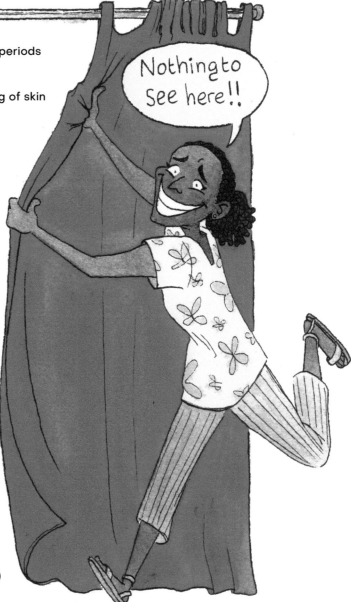

This list isn't exhaustive, even if it's exhausting to read.

"Perimenopause... seems to exacerbate any existing condition or predisposition to certain things," says Maria Araujo; examples include allergies, hypothyroidism, fibromyalgia, and arthritis.[13] For those with a fine-tuned nervous system, the symptoms can be even more pronounced. This is a time when women need to pay extra attention to their health.

After menopause, most estrogen is manufactured in the body's fat cells (adipose tissue). An enzyme (aromatase) can convert other hormones into estrogen.[14]

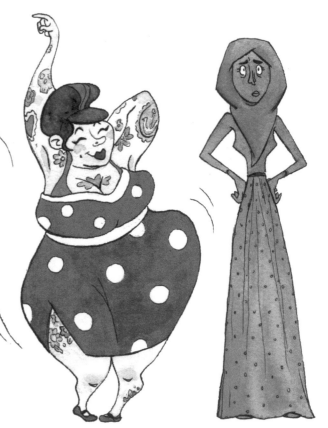

Thin women will likely suffer more than plump women because there is less availability of estrogen from fat stored in cells.[15] Estrogen contributes to cognitive health, bone health, the function of the cardiovascular system, and other essential bodily processes.

So, no dramatic dieting, ladies. Let the plump among us rejoice!

There are neurological symptoms of hormonal changes associated with natural and surgically induced menopause, in which the brain energy levels dip, and some women are at increased risk of Alzheimer's, according to Dr. Lisa Mosconi.[16] But wait! The microbiome has a huge impact on brain health; there are things you can do with what you choose to eat! More on this shortly.

"Hormone levels bouncing up and down ...in [a] frantic response to desperate signals from the brain to the pituitary, her menstrual cycle not only becomes erratic, but is uncoupled from her temperature and sleep cycles, and affects her appetite, sexual interest, and overall sense of well-being. The body's whole balance is thrown off. ... unsettling... but it is a temporary phenomenon, and one should not be [pushed] into a hysterectomy or onto hormones."

- Gail Sheehy[17]

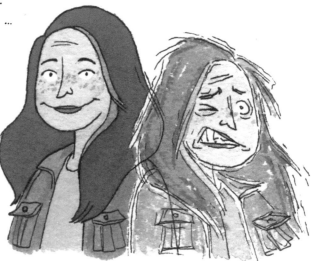

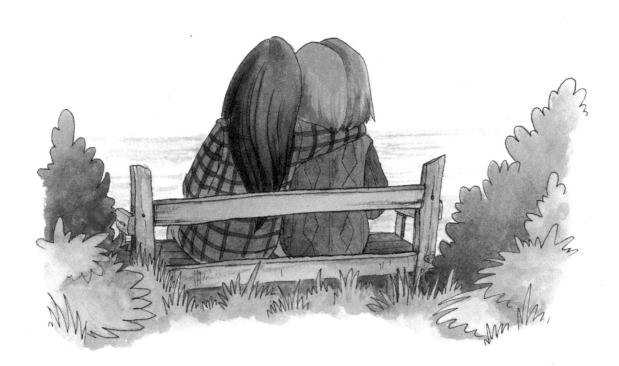

EARLY 40S

Let's take a moment away from humor. No proven link exists between depression and menopause. Yet 80% of menopausal women self-report feelings of nervousness and irritability.[18] While the state is temporary and feelings of sadness are not the same as DSM-III criteria for depression, sad feelings should not be trivialized.

Women's responsibilities can be heavy at this age. They may be raising children, caring for aging parents, working, and without enough help (healthcare, childcare, money, time). Perimenopausal symptoms exacerbate the mess.

I have observed a significant number of women in their early 40s suffering, and the outcomes can be damaging. Drug addiction, cheating, divorce, and all kinds of other self-destructive behaviors can arise. My former obstetrician declared that most of her patients were on antidepressant drugs, and why shouldn't I be? A carefully guided approach to pharmaceuticals has a helpful place in care; this does not mean numbing all women in their 40s! My concern is that women are being rushed there, in lieu of a holistic plan supporting overall health.

Be careful and seek help. Talk to a therapist if you can. A healthy approach includes eating well enough, moderate exercise, practicing good mental health techniques, including pharmaceutical support if necessary, and fostering supportive human connections. This is hard and essential work.

MENOPAUSE AND DISABILITIES

I like humor. As the saying goes, if I don't laugh, I'll cry! Still, I must set the humor aside for one more page. I offer no solutions, only awareness here.

If you happen to be disabled, you probably know that matters are even worse than for those who don't carry that burden.

If a woman is disabled, counselors, friends, and doctors do not typically talk about any subject that is considered "sexual." This includes talking about menstruation and menopause. According to Shirley Masuda, from the Disabled Women's Network, this is called "disability castration syndrome."[19] It results in a critical lack of research funding to yield essential information to support this already vulnerable group.

If pre-existing conditions can be worsened with the rapid changes in hormones associated with perimenopause, this can be particularly challenging for individuals who may be navigating already complex medical needs. Managing the medical support of disabilities can be complex to begin with, never mind trying to do it with a complete lack of support from good research, a supportive medical community, and a body going out of sync with itself. There are many examples one could explore in this vast field. For instance, multiple sclerosis patients are sensitive to heat; adding hot flashes into the mix is problematic.[20]

I remain hopeful that advocates for the disabled can shine a light in this area too.

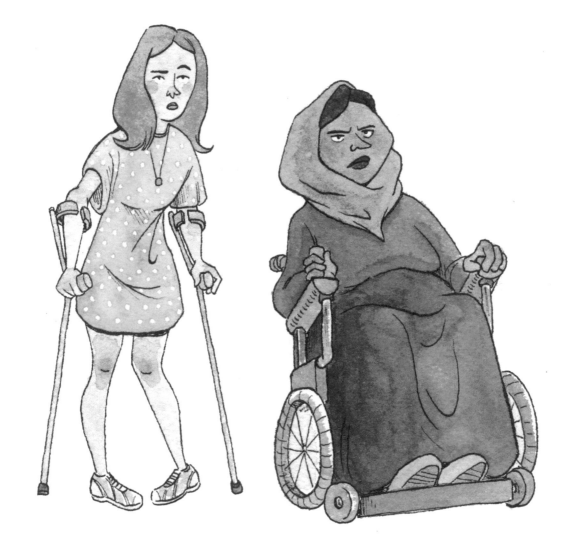

Disabled women facing perimenopause are offered little information or support, a problem for those managing intersecting symptoms.

WHAT YOU CAN DO (THE SHORT LIST)

EAT WELL! Avoid (reduce?!) processed foods. Organic foods support a healthy gut.[21]

AVOID STRENUOUS DIETING. Most estrogen post-menopause is from fat cells.

BE METHODICAL. Use coping skills to manage temporary memory loss. (If you can remember to.)

EXERCISE. Yes, groan. But it's true.

ESTROGEN SUPPLEMENTS. Maintain bone in the early years of menopause.

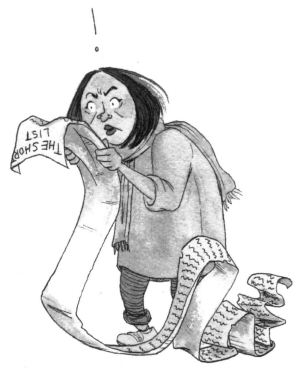

LOW DOSE VAGINAL MEDICATION. Treat vaginal dryness (it's not the end of your sex life!).

HEART HEALTH. Cardiovascular disease kills off one in two women over 50.

HORMONES. See warnings, please.

NATURAL SUPPLEMENTS WebMD lists Black Cohosh (hot flashes), Flaxseed (night sweats), Calcium and Vitamin D (bone loss), Ginseng (sleep, mood), St John's Wort (mood swings), and Soy (hot flashes).[22] Ask your OBGYN for products that support multiple symptoms. Supplements can have side effects, interfere with other medicines, or cause allergic reactions; consult your doctor.

You survived puberty and maybe pregnancy too. In either case, your body changed, and you had to manage your health. You can do this!

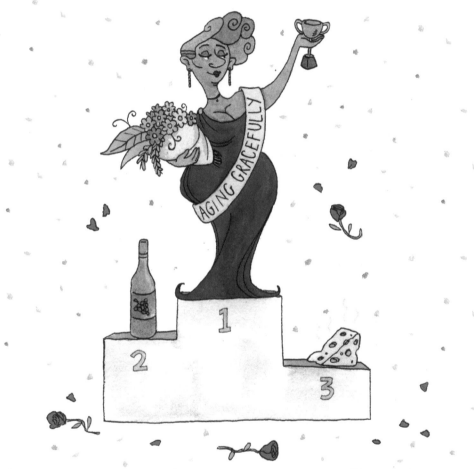

"Despite the trial-and-error state of medical care, a woman at fifty now has a second chance. To use it, she must make an alliance with her body and negotiate with her vanity. Today's healthy, active pacesetters will become the pioneers, mapping out a whole new territory for potent living and wisdom-sharing from one's fifities to one's eighties and even beyond."

-- Gail Sheehy[23]

THOSE DEVILISH DETAILS

Hormone replacement therapy is the "largest uncontrolled clinical trial in the history of medicine," according to Dr. Lewis Kuller.[24] Hormone therapy must be individualized. According to Professor Barbara Sherwin, no two women respond the same way, and the first year is trial and error. Nasty side effects (heart disease, breast cancer) can be experienced, especially if you are on hormones too long.[25]

Surgery can be necessary (e.g., removal of benign or malignant tumors, stubborn urogynecological conditions, treatment of problems related to fertility or ectopic pregnancy). However, taking the ovaries or uterus has been shown to increase the risk of dementia in women, according to Dr. Mosconi.[26] (Okay, this sucks, and I'm sorry. Please keep reading for what you can specifically do to support your brain.)

Brain health! Eat foods high in omega-3-fatty acids and antioxidants and phytoestrogen (cold-water fatty fish like salmon, trout, herring, anchovies, sardines), which reduce the risk of hormonal depression. Eat berries (cherries, blueberries, blackberries, goji -- all high in vitamin C) and good quality dark chocolate (theobromine, which has a similar effect to caffeine), which stimulates blood flow in the brain, slowing cellular aging. Follow a Mediterranean diet to lower the risk of cardiovascular disease, diabetes, obesity, breast cancer, and dementia in women. Eat apricots, strawberries, melon, watermelon, chickpeas, flax seeds, soy (phytoestrogen), and Brazil Nuts (Selenium).[27]

Avoid commercially grown, non-organic foods (vegetables and animals). You are putting xenoestrogens into your body that disrupt your natural estrogen, essentially competing with your own hormones.[28] (This is bad.)

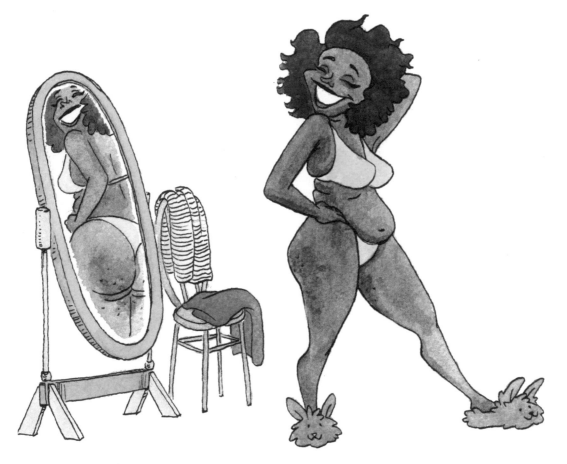

"If you look after yourself and you're healthy, then you'll have the energy to do things. But not to recognize getting older for what it is? I do think the infantilization of our generation is one of the huge issues of our time. People wanting to be 35 when they're 50 makes me think: Why? Why don't you be 50 and be good at that? And also embody the kinds of choices that are sustainable at that age."

- Emma Thompson[29]

GLASS HALF FULL

You are gasping, "Is there anything to look forward to?" Yes! Menopause will bring you a new state of equilibrium; energy, moods, overall physical and mental well-being should be restored.

Aging is not just a sad and empty decline. A recent study published in the journal Proceedings of the National Academy of Sciences has reported findings that women may be better positioned to learn later in life because their brains tend to be more youthful than their male counterparts.[30] Recent research shows that as we age, our brains change in ways that actually make us more positive. The emotional peak in life can occur in our 60s and 70s. Our values tend to shift, making us look more to giving back. We are living longer; these additional 10 to 15 years can be productive and happy. Innovation is not all from youth, as the media will have us believe; in fact, based on a study from the Census Bureau, the majority of successful businesses were founded by people over 50.[31]

The word menopause is about what is lost. Our periods stop... hmm, are we really complaining? I do not know too many (any?) women who are delighted come that time of the month. Menopause is a gateway to a second adulthood, it's a series of stages gifted to the very long-lived. Perhaps we could find a new word to capture what is gained, rather than what is lost.

"I suppose the time will never come when women, or men, either, will delight in crow's feet, wrinkles or grey hairs, but the time will come. . . when they will view these blemishes as but a petty price to pay for the joy of added wisdom, for the deeper joy of closer contact with humanity, and for the deepest joy of worthy work well done."

- Elizabeth Cady Stanton[32]

REFRAME

As you went through puberty (wasn't that fun?), you had to learn who you were, even in the midst of hormonal upheaval. You adjusted, you formed yourself. It's time to do that again. Just like puberty, you are on this train, and there is no getting off. You can achieve a new plateau of contentment and self-acceptance, with a broader view of the world and all the advantages of experience behind you. You can embrace the potential, a potent new burst of energy by mid-fifties.

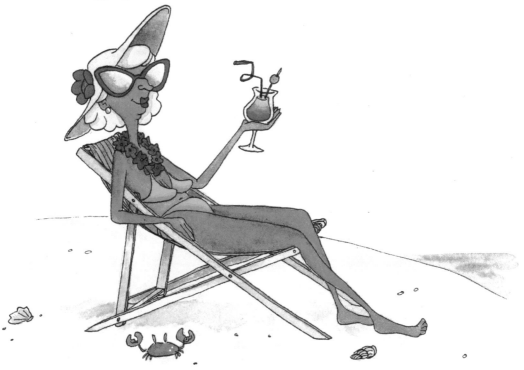

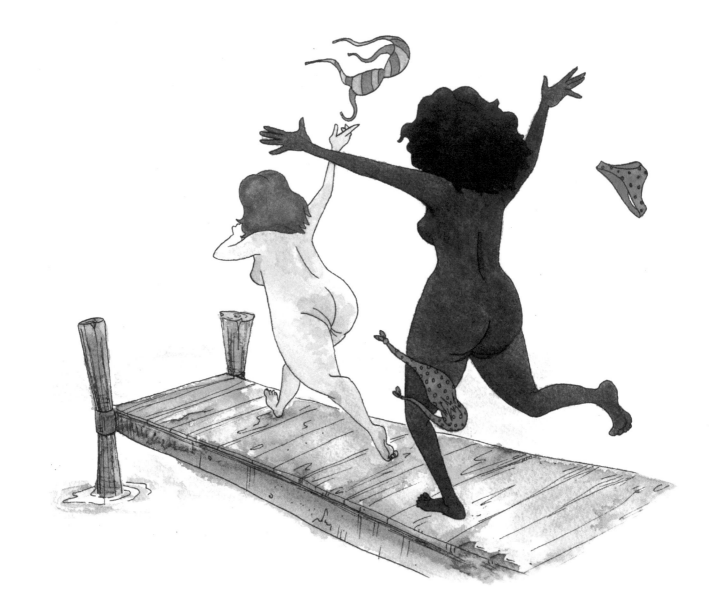

THERE. THAT WASN'T SO BAD, WAS IT?

What you're going through is part of the experience of living and growth. It beats the alternative, yes? And, if you need it, the consolation prize is that what is on the other side of this hormonally wild phase can be quite liberating and empowering.

SO!

TAKE CARE OF YOURSELF.

BE PATIENT.

LAUGH A LOT.

AND GOOD LUCK.

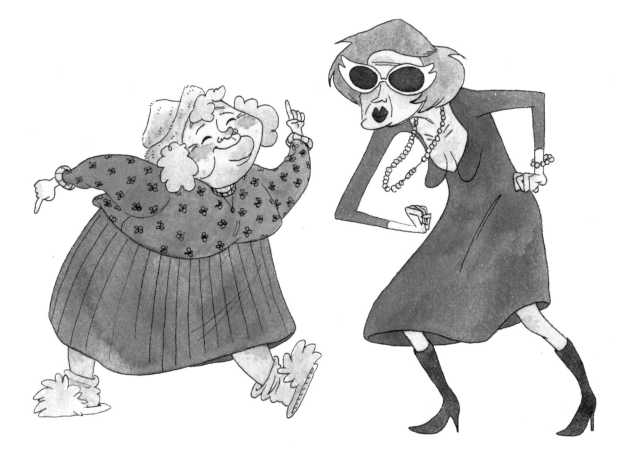

"There is a saying that with age, you look outside what you are inside. If you are someone who never smiles your face gets saggy. If you're a person who smiles a lot, you will have more smile lines. Your wrinkles reflect the roads you have taken; they form the map of your life."

- Diane von Furstenberg[33]

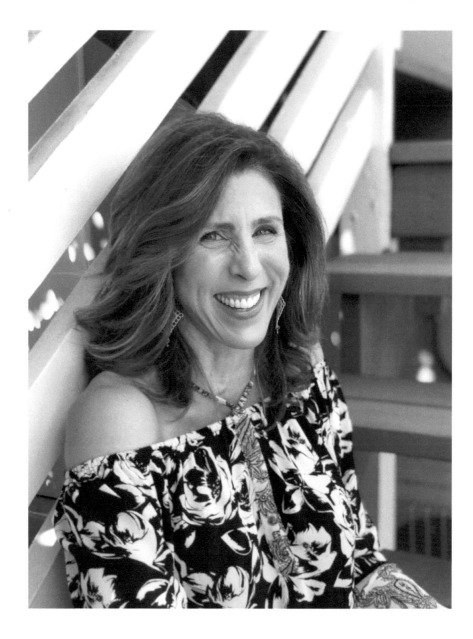

The Author

HEATHER WRIGHT is a Canadian located in the San Francisco Bay Area and is a first-time author. She has enjoyed terrific careers that use her fancy Master's degrees in Chemical Engineering and Fine Arts too. She has done odd things like get her name on a toner patent for Xerox and led a significant historical clock restoration project for Queen's University. Yet her only real credentials for writing this book are her enviable gender (female) and age (in her 40s). She wrote this book because, for goodness sake, someone had to.

www.whatshappeningtomenow.com
@whatshappeningtomenow

The Illustrator

MATYLDA MCCORMACK-SHARP is an Illustrator and a recent graduate of the Academy of Art University. Originally from the United Kingdom, Matylda now resides in the San Francisco Bay Area, pursuing a career in the arts. Matylda's excellence is well recognized. Her work has been featured in the competitive Academy of Arts Spring Show a few times, including a first-place award from the Graphic Novel and Motion Graphics and runner up for Children's Book Illustration categories. Although she has no menopausal experience, it is inevitable that one day she will. She illustrated this book because, for goodness sake, someone had to.

www.matyldamai.com
@matyldraws

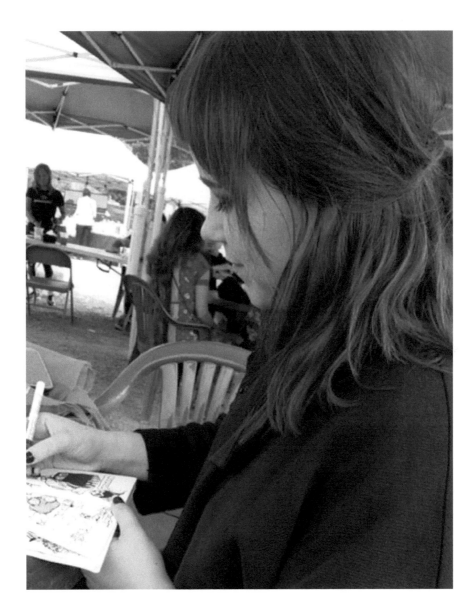

END NOTES

[1] Gail Sheehy, "The Silent Passage," Vanity Fair, last modified December 3, 2013, https://www.vanityfair.com/news/1991/10/menopause-politics-healthcare.

[2] Gail Sheehy, "The Silent Passage," Vanity Fair, last modified December 3, 2013, https://www.vanityfair.com/news/1991/10/menopause-politics-healthcare.

[3] Gail Sheehy, "The Silent Passage," Vanity Fair, last modified December 3, 2013, https://www.vanityfair.com/news/1991/10/menopause-politics-healthcare.

[4] Gail Sheehy, "The Silent Passage," Vanity Fair, last modified December 3, 2013, https://www.vanityfair.com/news/1991/10/menopause-politics-healthcare.

[5] Gail Sheehy, "The Silent Passage," Vanity Fair, last modified December 3, 2013, https://www.vanityfair.com/news/1991/10/menopause-politics-healthcare.

[6] GrrlScientist, "Invisible Women: Exposing Data Bias in A World Designed for Men," Forbes, accessed October 22, 2019, https://www.forbes.com/sites/grrlscientist/2019/10/22/invisible-women-exposing-data-bias-in-a-world-designed-for-men/#d4f72ff3989e.

[7] Laura Hambleton, "Primatologist Jane Goodall, 77, Talks About How Chimps and Humans Age," The Washington Post, last modified December 5, 2011, https://www.washingtonpost.com/national/health-science/primatologist-jane-goodall-77-talks-about-how-chimps-and-humans-age/2011/11/28/gIQAmA7DWO_story.html.

[8] Laura Hambleton, "Primatologist Jane Goodall, 77, Talks About How Chimps and Humans Age," The Washington Post, last modified December 5, 2011, https://www.washingtonpost.com/national/health-science/primatologist-jane-goodall-77-talks-about-how-chimps-and-humans-age/2011/11/28/gIQAmA7DWO_story.html.

[9] Gail Sheehy, "The Silent Passage," Vanity Fair, last modified December 3, 2013, https://www.vanityfair.com/news/1991/10/menopause-politics-healthcare.

[10] Gail Sheehy. "The Silent Passage," Vanity Fair, last modified December 3, 2013, https://www.vanityfair.com/news/1991/10/menopause-politics-healthcare.

[11] Dr. Jen Gunter, *The Vagina Bible* (New York: Citadel Press Kensington Publishing Corp, 2019), 159-160.

[12] Gail Sheehy, "The Silent Passage," Vanity Fair, last modified December 3, 2013, https://www.vanityfair.com/news/1991/10/menopause-politics-healthcare.

[13] Lynne Swanson, "Surviving the Change – Menopause and Women with Disabilities," Women with Disabilities Australia (WWDA), last modified Spring, 1998, http://wwda.org.au/issues/health/health1995/menop1/.

[14] Dr. Jen Gunter, *The Vagina Bible* (New York: Citadel Press Kensington Publishing Corp, 2019), 160.

[15] Dr. Jen Gunter, *The Vagina Bible* (New York: Citadel Press Kensington Publishing Corp, 2019), 160.

[16] Shannon Perry, "Menopause, Alzheimer's, & Eating for Retirement with Dr. Lisa Mosconi, Part 1," Gennev, accessed December 10, 2019,

https://gennev.com/menopause-alzheimers-estrogen/.

[17] Gail Sheehy, "The Silent Passage." Vanity Fair, December 3, 2013, https://www.vanityfair.com/news/1991/10/menopause-politics-healthcare.

[18] Gail Sheehy, "The Silent Passage." Vanity Fair, December 3, 2013, https://www.vanityfair.com/news/1991/10/menopause-politics-healthcare.

[19] Lynne Swanson, "Surviving the Change – Menopause and Women with Disabilities," Women with Disabilities Australia (WWDA), last modified Spring, 1998, http://wwda.org.au/issues/health/health1995/menop1/.

[20] Lynne Swanson, "Surviving the Change – Menopause and Women with Disabilities," Women with Disabilities Australia (WWDA), last modified Spring, 1998, http://wwda.org.au/issues/health/health1995/menop1/.

[21] Dr. Lisa Mosconi."Here's What Women Should Eat to Maintain a Healthy Brain," ideas.Ted.com, accessed March 11, 2020, https://ideas.ted.com/heres-what-women-should-eat-to-maintain-a-healthy-brain/.

[22] Dr. Traci C. Johnson, "Natural Treatments for Menopause Symptoms," WebMD, last modified August 4, 2018, https://www.webmd.com/menopause/guide/menopause-natural-treatments.

[23] Gail Sheehy, "The Silent Passage," Vanity Fair, last modified December 3, 2013, https://www.vanityfair.com/news/1991/10/menopause-politics-healthcare.

[24] Gail Sheehy, "The Silent Passage," Vanity Fair, last modified December 3, 2013, https://www.vanityfair.com/news/1991/10/menopause-politics-healthcare.

[25] Gail Sheehy, "The Silent Passage," Vanity Fair, last modified December 3, 2013, https://www.vanityfair.com/news/1991/10/menopause-politics-healthcare.

[26] Deborah Copaken, "Exploring the Link Between Menopause and Alzheimer's," Medium, accessed May 30, 2019, https://medium.com/neurotrack/menopause-and-alzheimers-1c455f29fe16.

[27] Dr. Lisa Mosconi."Here's What Women Should Eat to Maintain a Healthy Brain," ideas.Ted.com, accessed March 11, 2020, https://ideas.ted.com/heres-what-women-should-eat-to-maintain-a-healthy-brain/.

[28] Deborah Copaken, "Exploring the Link Between Menopause and Alzheimer's," Medium, accessed May 30, 2019, https://medium.com/neurotrack/menopause-and-alzheimers-1c455f29fe16.

[29] Julie Ma, "25 Famous Women on Getting Older," The Cut, last modified September 25, 2014, https://www.thecut.com/2014/09/25-famous-women-on-aging.html.

[30] Jon Hamilton, "Scans Show Female Brains Remain Youthful as Male Brains Wind Down," NPR All Things Considered, last modified February 4, 2019, https://www.npr.org/sections/health-shots/2019/02/04/691356272/scans-show-womens-brains-remain-youthful-as-male-brains-wind-down.

[31] Frank Olito, "8 Famous Companies Started by People in Their 50s and Older," Business Insider, accessed January 23, 2020, https://www.businessinsider.com/companies-started-middle-aged-50s-60s.

[32] Melissa Walker, "The Hey-day of Woman's Life: Elizabeth Cady Stanton and the Journey Toward Your Personal Heyday," Heyday Coaching, last modified August 22, 2016, https://www.heydaycoaching.com/blog/2016/8/22/the-hey-day-of-womans-life-elizabeth-cady-stanton-and-the-journey-toward-your-personal-heyday.

[33] Julie Ma, "25 Famous Women on Getting Older," The Cut, last modified September 25, 2014, https://www.thecut.com/2014/09/25-famous-women-on-aging.html.

[34] Alicia Cara, "Scars to Your Beautiful," track 10 on Know-It-All, Def Jam Recordings, 2015, compact disc.

BIBLIOGRAPHY

Cara, Alicia. "Scars to Your Beautiful." Track 10 on *Know-It-All*. Def Jam Recordings, 2015, compact disc.

Chen, Angela. "A Journalist Explains the Dangerous Consequences of a World Built for Men." The Verge. Last modified March 5, 2019. https://www.theverge.com/2019/3/5/18251570/caroline-criado-perez-invisible-women-data-bias-science-gender.

Copaken, Deborah. "Exploring the Link Between Menopause and Alzheimer's." Medium. Last modified May 30, 2019. https://medium.com/neurotrack/menopause-and-alzheimers-1c455f29fe16.

GrrlScientist, "Invisible Women: Exposing Data Bias in A World Designed for Men." Forbes. Accessed October 22, 2019. https://www.forbes.com/sites/grrlscientist/2019/10/22/invisible-women-exposing-data-bias-in-a-world-designed-for-men/#d4f72ff3989e.

Goldman, Rena. "10 Books That Shine a Light on Menopause." Healthline. Last modified July 12, 2017. https://www.healthline.com/health/menopause/best-menopause-books-of-the-year#1.

Gunter, Jen. *The Vagina Bible.* New York: Citadel Press Kensington Publishing Corp., 2019.

Hambleton, Laura. "Primatologist Jane Goodall, 77, Talks About How Chimps and Humans Age." The Washington Post. Last modified December 5, 2011. https://www.washingtonpost.com/national/health-science/primatologist-jane-goodall-77-talks-about-how-chimps-and-humans-age/2011/11/28/gIQAmA7DWO_story.html.

Harvard Women's Health Watch. "Why You Should Thank Your Aging Brain." Harvard Health Publishing. Last modified March 2015. https://www.health.harvard.edu/mind-and-mood/why-you-should-thank-your-aging-brain.

Johnson, Traci. "Natural Treatments for Menopause Symptoms." WebMD. Last modified August 4, 2018. https://www.webmd.com/menopause/guide/menopause-natural-treatments.

Ma, Julie. "25 Famous Women on Getting Older." The Cut. Last modified September 25, 2014. https://www.thecut.com/2014/09/25-famous-women-on-aging.html.

Olito, Frank. "8 Famous Companies Started by People in Their 50s and Older." Business Insider. Accessed January 23, 2020. https://www.businessinsider.com/companies-started-middle-aged-50s-60s.

Perry, Shannon. "Menopause, Alzheimer's, & Eating for Retirement with Dr. Lisa Mosconi, Part 1." Gennev. Last modified December 10, 2019. https://gennev.com/menopause-alzheimers-estrogen/.

Perry, Shannon. "Menopause, Alzheimer's, & Eating for Retirement with Dr. Lisa Mosconi, Part 2." Gennev. Last modified March 22, 2019. https://gennev.com/menopause-alzheimers-risk-part-2/.

Sheehy, Gail. "The Silent Passage." Vanity Fair. Last modified December 3, 2013. https://www.vanityfair.com/news/1991/10/menopause-politics-healthcare.

Swanson, Lynne. "Surviving the Change – Menopause and Women with Disabilities." Women with Disabilities Australia (WWDA). Last modified spring, 1998. http://wwda.org.au/issues/health/health1995/menop1/.

Mosconi, Lisa. "Here's What Women Should Eat to Maintain a Healthy Brain." ideas.Ted.com. Accessed March 11, 2020. https://ideas.ted.com/heres-what-women-should-eat-to-maintain-a-healthy-brain/.

Hamilton, Jon. "Hormone Levels Likely Influence a Woman's Risk of Alzheimer's, But How?" NPR All Things Considered. Last modified July 23, 2018. https://www.npr.org/sections/health-shots/2018/07/23/630688342/might-sex-hormones-help-protect-women-from-alzheimer-s-after-all-maybe.

Hamilton, Jon. "Scans Show Female Brains Remain Youthful as Male Brains Wind Down." NPR All Things Considered. Last modified February 4, 2019. https://www.npr.org/sections/health-shots/2019/02/04/691356272/scans-show-womens-brains-remain-youthful-as-male-brains-wind-down.

Walker, Melissa."The Hey-day of Woman's Life: Elizabeth Cady Stanton and the Journey Toward Your Personal Heyday." Heyday Coaching. Last modified August 22, 2016. https://www.heydaycoaching.com/blog/2016/8/22/the-hey-day-of-womans-life-elizabeth-cady-stanton-and-the-journey-toward-your-personal-heyday.

"You're beautiful just the way you are"

-- Alicia Cara, Scars to Your Beautiful[34]

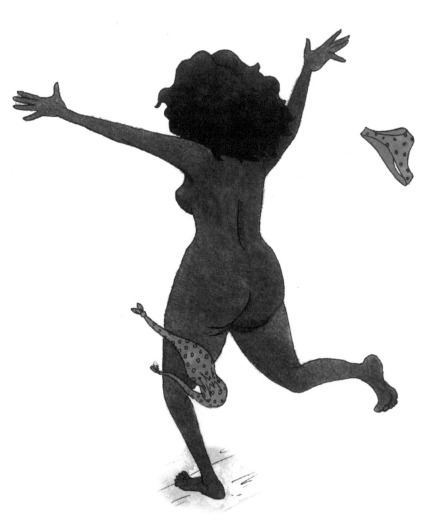

CPSIA information can be obtained
at www.ICGtesting.com
Printed in the USA
BVHW020508031120
592372BV00002B/7